BK RN

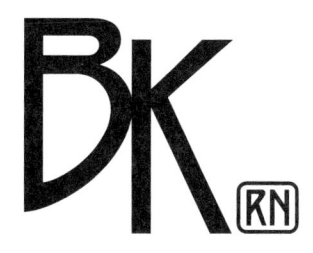

Knowledge Reduces Fear

VOL. 2

A RESOURCE FOR END OF LIFE EDUCATION

In Volume 1 of Knowledge Reduces Fear, I drew from my blog posts to lay a groundwork for understanding the natural dying process. Vol 2 addresses end of life areas I believe have misunderstanding attached to them.

The intent of both volumes is to provide knowledge about dying in an easy, non-threatening format that will ease some of the fear and misconceptions that we bring to this subject.

Blessings,

Barbara

Barbara Karnes, RN writes articles, answers questions and addresses concerns about end of life care on her award winning weekly blog - *Something to Think About: A Blog on End of Life*. Visit her website **bkbooks.com** to follow her blog and for more information about her work.

Table of Contents

Section I - Introduction
- The "Old Days" 1
- No One Dies Alone 3
- Hospice RN 4

Section II - Treatment
- Informed Choices 5
- What Are We Trying to Achieve? 6
- Cure, Remission, Shrinkage vs. Quality 7
- Miracles 8
- He Asked for Treatment 9
- Just Because We Can 10
- What to Do? 11

Section III - Food and Water
- It's Okay Not to Eat 13
- It's Okay Not to Drink Water 14
- Is it a Choice to Not Eat? 14
- Feeding Tube? 15

Section IV - Pain At End of Life
- Medications 16
- Morphine 17
- Lack of Knowledge 18
- Did Morphine Kill? 19
- The Patch 20
- Just Because They are Dying 21
- Help Me Die 22
- Guidelines 23

Section V - Children
- Coping 24
- Death Has No Age Limit 24
- Suicide 25
- Adult Children 26
- Miscarriage/Stillborn 26

Section VI - Faith
- Faith 28
- Non-Existence 29
- There are No Accidents 30

Section I: Memories

The Old Days

Someone recently asked me what hospice was like in the "old days." I felt a feeling similar to the one I had when my grandson asked me if there were cars when I was a kid.

In the "old days," hospice was different than it is now. Censuses were smaller, staff was smaller, average length of stay was in the range of 50 to 60 days. Our goal was to support and guide the family and patient through their final experience, and that included being with them at the time of death. Medical supplies and equipment were limited, as was our knowledge of pain management, or even of the actual dying process.

I started in the early '80s working for the first hospice in Kansas City. I was one of two RNs and between us we cared for 10 to 12 patients. We were supported by a chaplain, a social worker, and a volunteer coordinator. Both nurses saw all the patients, mostly alternating visits, sometimes visiting together.

We wanted the patients and families to have someone they knew to support and guide them through the challenging time: the moment of death. It was important that all the families knew, trusted, and had a relationship with both of us. The goblins always come at night so the other nurse and I alternated being on call (24/7 on, 24/7 off).

Our visits were scheduled based on the amount of time we thought the patient had to live. If we thought the patient had months, we visited once a week. If we judged they had weeks, then we visited two or three times a week. When it was days, we, of course, visited daily. If someone needed to be seen less than once a week then were they really appropriate for hospice?

If the person was close to death (hours to minutes) we stayed. I spent many nights on someone's sofa, or even the floor beside a bed, because the family was frightened and didn't want to be alone. If the person died or had signs of imminent death, they called us. We went to the home and stayed until the funeral home had come and gone. That was a good time to talk about funeral services, and about writing a letter, or drawing a picture to put in the casket. It gave us the opportunity to clean the room the patient had died in and set up a small memento on the pillow so the room would be peaceful when the family returned to it.

As I write, these memories are surfacing:

I remember a woman who wanted to go to Las Vegas to gamble one last time. I took her to the airport and when I picked her up on her return home, she told me she had never left her hotel room.

I remember dressing up in a Halloween costume every Halloween and visiting all of our patients and families. I wore the same costume every year: mother nature with a fairy wand. The families loved it. Yes, I probably looked silly. But we shared smiles.

I remember sleeping on a living room sofa because the family was afraid to be alone when Mom died. Death seemed imminent and yet she didn't die.

I suggested everyone tell her how much they loved her one more time and go to bed. I said she may want privacy or to protect them. I would stay on the sofa in the next room and go to sleep also.

One daughter said "Mom can't die alone. I will sit with her". It was agreed she would stay but everyone else would go to sleep, which we did. At some point in the early morning the daughter woke me to say she had fallen asleep and awakened to find her mother dead.

We all gathered around the bed and said our goodbyes again. I called the funeral home and, when the body was gone, said my goodbyes, telling them I would see them at the visitation.

I remember crawling in bed and holding a woman in my arms as we talked about how afraid she was to die.

I remember eating a piece of custard pie that a woman insisted I eat every time I visited her husband. It was the same pie, and it sat on the kitchen counter all week. By the end of the week I was a bit concerned about the state of that pie but she was so proud of it, and the ability to thank me for coming, that I ate every bite. He died about the same time the pie was finished.

I remember using handmade bed pads from a place called Cancer Action. Volunteers sewed old sheets around newspaper. We used Udder Ointment for skin care and mayonnaise jars for urinals. We were among the first to use Elizabeth Kuebler Ross's Brompton Cocktail for pain management which allowed the patient to control the schedule and dosage. Patient controlled pain relief! What a radical act that was!!

I remember a doctor not allowing me to turn off the ventilator a patient with ALS was on until he, the doctor, came to the house to pronounce the man dead. The family and I sat in the beloved man's room for hours wondering how we would know when he was actually dead, since he would still be breathing. We watched his body turn purple, not sure if there was a faint pulse or not, getting no blood pressure. At some point the room just felt different. I can't describe it, but it was then we knew he was gone. The physician eventually came to the house to turn off the machine.

What a difference it is today. Back then we had months to get to know the patient and family. As a result of primary care nursing, bonding and trust developed. We didn't have to deal with "wage and hour", or medicare's micromanaging, or fear of insurance claims. We were basically outside of the medical model giving supportive, nurturing care as a person died. We learned as we went. There weren't classes on how to care for end of life situations. We learned, then we shared, then we taught.

No One Dies Alone

Dear Barbara, I am a hospice volunteer and am occasionally with a patient when family members are unavailable to be with a person as they near their death. Of course this is a sad situation for the dying person being alone as they leave this world. Sometimes I arrive to find that family members or friends have arrived. My question is, how can I best support these people at this highly emotional time? I generally let them know that we are there to help if needed and offer to sit in their place if they need to make phone calls or get something to eat. I remind them that they can always call if they need anything else. I then usually take my leave and give them their privacy. But I wonder if there is something else I should say or do that might help? Is it appropriate to ask about their dying relative? Is it helpful for them to speak about the person or is it better just to let the family be with their own thoughts?

When I was doing direct patient care in the '80s our hospice goal was to be with the family at the patient's moment of death. The hours before actual death are very scary, an "I don't know what to do" time, for anyone present. Someone who knows the normal, natural way a person dies can be like a conductor as they guide those present through the experience. You being there with your knowledge of end of life can have a significant role in turning an often frightening time into a sacred one. So, yes, I think you should stay if people unexpectedly arrive. Explain that if it is alright, you would like to stay and be of assistance. Most people will welcome your presence.

I would like to see hospice programs offer trained volunteers to every family, not just to those patients that have no family. The person who is actively dying is like a little chicken trying to get out of its shell, working very hard. They are so removed from their physical body that their attention is inward, not outward, so actually whether they are alone or have a room full of people isn't the important issue. The real need is to provide support to the family and significant others who are there with the person who is actively dying. It is those who are present that need guidance.

Even though the dying person is busy they can still hear, so with that in mind, here are some suggestions for working with the family:
- Explain to everyone about the "little chick" idea. This gives them a base line for understanding what is happening. You want them to know that nothing bad is occurring. This is how people die and their special person is doing a good job. I often explain the days to hours before death as labor, the labor that precedes a birth into another world.
- Once you have neutralized the fear of what is happening, suggest that each person there spend time alone, talking with the one dying. Life is full of positive and negative occurrences. The person who is dying is processing their life so help them by talking about the good and the difficult times.
- Tell the family that they can touch, hold, crawl in bed, cuddle. They can laugh, cry, sing, reminisce. No need for quiet, the lights dimmed, or shades drawn.
- Help those present say goodbye. Because we have limited control over the time that we die suggest that the family tell their special person "when you are ready you can go". This is not to say that it is okay but that there is an understanding that their person is leaving.

Hospice RN

QUESTION: *Do you have any advice to provide a new hospice RN? It would be greatly appreciated! After working in several areas of nursing, I truly feel that hospice is my calling, and I want to do it right.*

Welcome to the world of hospice nursing and congratulations on finding your special place. So few find their special place anymore. For too many workers their job is just a job with a paycheck. How lucky you are to have found both.

I don't know about advice but I'll give you something to think about. My philosophy is that end of life care is not about medical interventions, treatments, procedures, pills or morphine. End of life care is about teaching, guidance, support and nurturing. It is about reassuring the family that nothing bad is happening, that their loved one is doing exactly what a person who is dying does, and that they are doing a good job. End of life care is all about neutralizing the fear everyone brings to this experience, the family and the patient.

How do we neutralize fear? By teaching the normal process of dying to the family, by encouraging the family in the care they are giving, by being available, by bonding with the family. Only by bonding with the family can you earn their trust to guide them through this uncomfortable experience. (That is why having primary care nursing is vital in hospice nursing. Families can't trust if every nurse they see is different, which is happening in way too many agencies.)

Your key teaching areas will be around eating and not eating. Explain why the body doesn't want the food. Do the same with hydration. Being dehydrated is just going to sleep and not waking up; all normal and part of the natural process. You will teach mouth and skin care, bowel management. Explain how the patient is withdrawing and sleeping more. Of course, if pain is an issue teach how we are the experts in pain and comfort management and why addiction and overdosing is not going to happen.

Remember that dying is not painful. It is disease that causes pain so if pain is not part of the disease history there is no need for morphine at end of life.

If you teach your families well about the approaching end of life, there will be no problems with them understanding the labor of dying. Having someone you care about dying is very sad but it doesn't have to be a bad experience. It is our job to see that their experience is a sacred one.

Section II: Treatment

Informed Choices

Generally speaking, a person goes to a physician because something is amiss with their physical body. We don't feel well so we go to doctors for help. Physicians "fix" what ails us. That is their job. We expect to receive some kind of treatment to make us better. Maybe we will get pills, maybe tests and procedures, or blood/lab work will be required but eventually the physician will tell us what is physically wrong with our bodies and what we need to do to return to our regular, non sick, life.

Unfortunately, our visit to the doctor doesn't always work out that way. Sometimes the report following all the tests and procedures is that it is going to be difficult to fix this one. We are going to try but the odds are not with us.

What do we do now becomes the big question? What odds are being talked about? Is it a cure that we are aiming for, remission or just more time? What will the side effects of the treatment be vs. the length of time we are hoping for with the treatment? How am I going to feel with treatment, without treatment? Are good days worth trading for the bad ones? All these questions are important to the decisions we will make. Yet most people don't ask the questions. Most people just look at their physician, or group of physicians, and blindly go in the direction they are pointed.

Blindly is the operative word here. Most of us don't ask the necessary questions to make informed choices. Why? Because doctors are supposed to care for us, be concerned about what is best for us, and help us be the best we can be physically.

I think that once upon a time that may have been the case. We had a family physician who often birthed us into this world and was at our bedside when we died (or the physician's son was there when we died). Remember Marcus Welby MD? Well those days, except maybe in very rural areas, are gone.

Now we have specialists, we have clinics with multiple physicians, we have emergency walk-in care centers and emergency rooms. And all these care centers mean less personal interactions, less knowing the patient. Healthcare has become more about knowing the disease, the illness, and less about the patient.

We, who receive this kind of healthcare, need to become proactive, to ask questions, do our own research. Google has opened a world of knowledge to us. Let's use it. With knowledge of our disease, the disease process, treatment options, side effects and success rates we can ask pertinent questions and take an active role in our partnership with physicians. We can choose treatments based on fact or choose no treatment, again, based on research not emotions and fear. Knowledge reduces fear.

With increased knowledge we also want a second opinion. Not from a doctor recommended by the one who gave us the original diagnosis, not from one in the same clinic. You want a second opinion from a physician who is not associated with the same neighborhood or hospital as the first physician. This is not being disloyal. It is about making informed decisions. We price shop for big financial purchases. We quality shop for home renovation and purchasing cars. It doesn't make sense that we would blindly accept one person's choice of treatment when our life depends on the decisions made —but we often do.

What Are We Trying To Achieve?

QUESTION: *What are we trying to achieve with treatment?*

That is THE question everyone involved in medical decision making needs to ask. Who is everyone? Physician, patient, and family.

Most people (patients and family) faced with an illness look for the treatment to cure them; to return them to our life as it was before the illness occurred. However, with today's medical accomplishments, fixing or curing may not be the only goal. Keeping the person alive, even if quality of life is sacrificed greatly, may be the medical goal. But is it the patient's goal? We need to ask. Yet most of us don't. We just assume our physician is thinking the same way we are.

What questions do we need to ask and consider to ensure that all involved are working in harmony toward the same goal?

"Can my illness be cured?" If you have a broken leg you can be pretty sure your goal and your physician's are the same--to get you walking again. If you have cancer, you might be expecting the physician to make it go away and return you to your normal life. Your physician may be expecting to slow your tumor growth or shrink its size a bit, but not cure you. See the difference?

"Can my illness be put into remission if a cure isn't possible? What are the chances the proposed treatment can put the disease process into remission? What about inhibiting further progression? What about tumor shrinkage? These are all pertinent questions we need to ask when we are looking at any particular treatment options.

"Just how sick am I going to be with the treatment? What are all of the side effects?" The gains of a particular treatment may not be worth the debilitation caused by its medications and side effects. Sometimes we've only added two weeks to a pain filled life at the cost of three months of agonizing, incapacitating side effects.

Remember, we are more than a physical body, we are emotional, mental, and spiritual. What are we doing for those parts of us when we pursue treatments without really understanding what we are getting ourselves into or what the expected outcome is? Are we headed for comfort or discomfort? Will the rest of our days be filled with illness and possibly pain?

Will the discomfort be worth the final outcome? Absolutely, if a cure is expected. Probably, if remission or even significantly slowing progression is expected. But if with the proposed treatment we will have a difficult time with maintaining the disease status quo, let alone fixing it, then is it worth it?

There is no right or wrong answer to all these questions. Some people will want to do every possible thing to live just a few more days, no matter the condition of the physical body. Others will want to take the time and live the best they can without medical intervention (except for pain management).

If the patient can't ask the questions (due to dementia or unconsciousness) that in itself can be an answer regarding body functioning and quality of life activities and the pursuit of treatments.

We can't make choices that are best for us if we don't have honest, accurate information upon which to base our decisions. We need to ask questions! We need to do our research! The Internet is a wonderful tool. It can help us get unbiased information. It has put a world of knowledge literally at our fingertips. Knowledge is power, knowledge reduces fear, and knowledge helps us make good decisions.

Cure, Remission, Shrinkage vs. Quality

QUESTION: *Please write about bargaining—the patient (with terminal brain cancer) trying to find a cure; trying to find holistic cures to save his life and spending whatever "extra" cash he has to do it.*

You've just described most people who have been told they have a life threatening illness. My question is "Why do we search for every possible avenue to stay alive when often we really aren't living life to its fullest in the first place?" Are most of us really living life when we are healthy let alone when we are sick?

Part of our inability to stop searching and trying "everything possible to keep us alive" begins with the medical professionals; their honesty, their forthrightness, the manner in which they present the diagnosis and treatment options to us. Unfortunately, this is not always done in a manner that tells us truthfully what the next year or six months of our life will be like and that death, not cure will be the ultimate outcome.

As I have written before, there is a huge difference between treatment for life threatening diseases and cure. Most people are willing to go through immense pain and difficulty for a cure and appropriately so, but most treatments for a lot of cancers may shrink the tumors but still leave a person incapacitated and dying.

It is generally not human nature to just lay down and die particularly with the medical advances we have made in the last century. Death used to be recognized as a part of living; a person got sick and then they died if they didn't get killed by the many events in their hard life first. Now we look at death as a failure in the medical system, not a natural course of events. Doctors are supposed to "fix" us and if one can't then we search for one who will.

I believe we all have the responsibility to try to be cured if our condition is curable. With the advent of the Internet and search engines we can research our condition, learn about our disease and with enough information decide if or how much treatment will make a difference. Armed with knowledge we can make informed choices; choices not based on fear, ignorance, and that innate drive to stay alive.

Added to the above opinion I think a person's personality is also an important player in these decisions. As an example, I think I have a low pain tolerance and probably avoid discomfort more than most people. My personality is such that I would not go for extensive treatments and medical procedures.

My step father, however, chose, because of the nature of his personality (a doer, in charge, very mental—not that all people with these personality characteristics will make the same choice), to undergo extensive treatments for his cancer, knowing the outcome was not favorable. Neither of these choices are a right or wrong way to face a serious, life threatening illness.

If we can get realistic facts about cure vs. remission vs. shrinkage and what those outcomes mean in relation to our quality of living, we can then make decisions based on knowledge.

We will all be afraid to some degree as we approach the end of our life. We will all be frightened to let go of the known for the unknown. No one wants to leave that which they know, even if living is difficult and challenging each day. My hope is that with honesty from the medical profession we can make informed decisions about how we want to live until we are dead, that we will not choose out of ignorance and fear to chase the unreachable.

Miracles

QUESTION: *Can you write about "miracles" and how the hope/prayer for a miracle can make people miss what is in front of them?*

The dictionary defines "miracle" as: "An event not explicable by natural or scientific laws. Such an event may be attributed to a supernatural being (God or gods), a miracle worker, a saint or a religious leader." With that definition you have to be a pretty high stakes gambler to bet your life (literally) on the idea that a miracle is going to cure your life threatening illness.

"People miss what is in front of them." That is a powerful statement. What is in front of us is the present, whatever the situation our life is in at the moment. What many, maybe even most, people do is trade that moment for a gamble on the future. We do this gambling with a lot of life occurrences. But we place our biggest bets with life threatening illness decisions.

We gamble that being very sick with side effects, and spending inordinate amounts of money on treatments and procedures, will result in a cure; in a life that is active and healthy, in a miracle. I use the word "miracle" because if the right questions are asked and the physician is being honest, often times the answers will point to this: it would take a miracle to return you to a healthy life. Most of us just don't want to hear that kind of answer, so we don't ask.

I remember someone telling me that prayer requires action, that God works through us. There is an old story about a man praying to God to save him from the rising waters of a river. A boat comes by and the driver says to the man "Get aboard." The man replies "God will save me." A rescue helicopter throws down a rope and the pilot says "Climb the rope." The man says " God will save me." Well, the man drowned. When he met God the man was disillusioned and asked God why he didn't save him. God replied "I tried. I sent you a boat and a helicopter." The point is clear. God's help comes in the ways of this earth. It is God working through us and our actions that creates miracles.

I think prayer/positive thinking is a very valuable tool in healing; in all of living actually, but it isn't enough. To deal with our challenges we must use the tools of the physical world we live in: rational thinking, research, and knowledge of our disease.

He Asked For Treatment

QUESTION: *I am having a very difficult time providing care for my father as a critical care nurse. I almost lost him to pneumonia. My agency insisted he not be treated and taking him to the ER would cause them to revoke hospice. He was treated with Levaquin and his quality of life is much improved. Who is right? Treat an infection or just let him die? He asked for treatment.*

The operative words here are "He asked for treatment." There is your answer. Our responsibility as health care workers, and I will argue that it is also the responsibility of family, is to provide what treatment or lack of treatment a person wants; to respect how a person wants to live and how a person wants to die. That is why Advance Directives are so important. It tells everyone what you want if you can't speak for yourself; and it also reaffirms what you want even when you can speak for yourself.

The problems (and there are several) generally lie in a person not having an Advanced Directive, in people thinking they know what is best for others, and with family members not reconciling with the approaching death. There is also a problem with healthcare professionals concentrating on keeping a body breathing (treating physical conditions) and not looking at the person, the suffering caused, and for what end the treatment is being done.

When a person accepts the Hospice Medicare Benefit it is because the person is physically at a place in their disease that cure is no longer considered possible; that in a physician's opinion the person has less than 6 months to live and that the patient is interested in comfort care for the family and themselves. They have accepted the notion that treatment is not the best option in addressing their physical condition. These circumstances and Medicare regulations put a Hospice agency in the position of having to say if you go to the ER and seek treatment you will not be eligible for Hospice services. Hospice is bound by Medicare Hospice regulations and rules.

The philosophy of Hospice end of life care is to assist those people who have reached a point in their disease process that cure is no longer possible. The philosophy is to provide comfort to the patient and support to the family during the last months and through the last hours of life. Therefore, if treatment is sought (treatment that will possibly prolong life), the person is considered not appropriate for Hospice services.

Now, with all this said, there are thin lines and points to debate. What is treatment to get better and treatment for comfort? Is pneumonia related to a life threatening illness or is it a separate disease not related to the condition that is the cause of approaching death? Is pneumonia really a very gentle way to die and the "old man's friend" as so many say?

What we do know is pneumonia left untreated in the frail will probably result in death. If a person is dying (they are on Hospice therefore considered to be dying) and they develop a condition that may result in death, what is the advantage in treating that condition? I have seen legs amputated and heart surgery done in people with severe life threatening illness unrelated to the surgeries. "Why" has always been my question. What was accomplished in doing surgery to amputate a leg or perform open heart surgery on a person with end stage cancer other than further suffering? These two incidents actually hastened death along with increasing the suffering.

So back to your question of treatment or no treatment as end of life approaches---the right answer is to do what the patient wants done. It is not really for the family or the physician to decide. It is the patient's choice. Confusion comes when no one knows what the person wants and they can't speak for themselves.

Just Because We Can

QUESTION: *The patient with bulbar onset ALS, a feeding tube, and unable to even speak. My mom.*

I'm not sure what the question is so I am going to interpret it as uncertainty as to what the future holds.

ALS is a horrific disease, not that there is a "good" disease but ALS traps a good mind in a slowly deteriorating, non functioning body affecting not only the ability to move all body parts but affects the ability to swallow (inability to eat) and the ability to breathe by themselves. See the movie based on Stephen Hawking's life, The Theory of Everything.

100 years ago when a person couldn't eat or breathe, they died. In our medical basket of tools today we can artificially feed someone who can't swallow and we can breathe for someone who can't make their chest muscles go up and down, in and out. The question now becomes "What do we do?" Just because we CAN do a medical procedure does that mean we SHOULD do it?

The thing is, even when we interrupt the natural dying process, death still comes because the disease still progresses. However, the timetable and signs of approaching death become less predictable.

The signs of approaching death from disease that begin months before death are: decrease in eating, increase in sleep, and gradual withdrawal emotionally and mentally from surroundings.

Artificial feeding (TPN, gastrostomy tube feeding, NG tube feeding) has complications but the body gets its nourishment and remains anchored to this planet. With artificial feeding, food intake is no longer a gauge to predict approaching death.

It is hard to keep people awake, so as death from disease begins to approach you will notice a person sleeping more and more. This is something you will look for and monitor, even when the person is getting artificial feeding.

We can't really affect a person's interest in the world around them so again, as death approaches, a person will continue to withdraw and be less interested in activities and happenings around them. Use their social interactions to help you determine if they are entering the dying process.

You can see that life for a person with ALS hinges on food, water, breathing and heart pumping and that will mean eventual artificial feeding and artificial breathing.

The mind of a person with ALS will still be sharp and alert before the dying process has begun but what about the emotions? What about the frustration of being trapped in a prison of a body, the anger, the helplessness, the sense of purpose or loss of it? Read Jojo Moyes book, Me Before You.

These challenges must be lived with and for some the choice of not having a feeding tube is a means of letting the disease run its course.

When the chest muscles can no longer make the pressure and movement to create an intake and output of oxygen another decision can be made; respirator/ventilator or none.

Is life worth living with all this assistance or not? For some it will be, for others it won't.

Today, with our medical technology, we can keep a body alive long after it ceases to be functional. Some people will choose to accept all the opportunities the medical profession can offer. "Keep my body going no matter how you have to do it!" Others will choose to have ventilators or respirators while others will stop at no artificial feeding. Some will choose nothing at all.

All are based on choices of what life and its quality personally means. There is no right or wrong answer to these different choices (This is where families and outsiders get confused, thinking their choice for another is the right choice).

Advanced Directives are important for all of us but particularly important for someone with ALS. When you can, make the decisions before they need to be made.

Just because we can do something medically doesn't mean it is the right choice to make. The right choice is the person's individual choice based on their personality and philosophy of living. It is a loving and sometimes difficult act to carry out a person's will for themselves after they have lost the ability to self advocate; especially when it is a different choice than we would have made for them.

What To Do

QUESTION: *I would like to know if my mother died at home, could we wash and care for her, and dress her for bed? Can a person have family come in and say their good byes? My sister thinks the body turns black and blows up and stinks up the house forever. My mother is 100 years old. She had a great life, and now that she is in pain, she wants to get out of this world. I am sure my sister's fears are not right. I would like her to die in her own bed, not alone in a hospital. I was reading about dying and from what you said, my mother was on her way out of this world very peacefully, when my sister took her to the hospital and put her on IV for seven days. Yes, she is back but she still can't eat or drink much. She is going to physical therapy to get stronger, so she can come home. I think no matter what we put this dear woman through, death is coming. The doctor said her body is healthy. Can a healthy body die if she doesn't eat or drink much? Should we engage her in exercise, even though she says she is tired? Are we putting her through all this exercise program for nothing in the end? She is 100 years old, maybe she just wants to sleep. Is that wrong? Will she die sooner if we don't wake her up and engage with her? I don't know what to do.*

I appreciate your thought out questions and the dilemma you are facing. The majority of our healthcare workers have not yet learned that just because you can do something medically doesn't mean it is in the best interest of the patient to do it. In my opinion this is one of those times. To put your mother through all of the medical procedures, IV's, hospitalizations and rehab seems a misinterpretation of "Do no harm" that is a physician's oath.

As you mentioned, what is wrong with letting your mother stay in her own home, own bed, own familiar surroundings, own routine? Nothing, as far as I can see. Her quality of life is affected with pain and the diminished capacities of her age. Peace and familiarity is her best medicine now. Let her eat what she wants or doesn't want, sleep when she wants to or doesn't want to, engage with her surroundings when she chooses. Let her life unfold as it will without medical intervention. Let you and your sister's gift to your mom be a gentle, natural death in the surroundings she is familiar with.

I would suggest that you ask your mom what she wants. It is her life so she needs to be making the decision of how to live it. If she is unable to communicate her wishes I see that as a sign in itself as to the quality of her life.

The question then becomes what are you and your sister wanting to achieve by putting your mother through the discomfort and disruption to her normal routine? Are you extending her bodily functions at the expense of her comfort? Is her body breathing but her mind not really interacting? If there are mental and emotional connections on her part, what are they?

These are all questions for you and your sister to explore. Sometimes we just want our mom here on this planet with us no matter the quality of life she has. Selfish, yes, but oh so normal.

In regard to your question about keeping your mother in your home after her death, there are state regulations and your funeral home can answer any of your questions. I believe it is appropriate for you to wash your mother's body, dress her and have family come to the house and say goodbye. Hug and kiss her body, crawl in bed with her and be close if you want, all before you call the funeral home. You do not need to have a service in church or a funeral home. You can say your goodbyes at home.

Now, timing is a factor in doing this. The body will start to get stiff in a few hours so you need to dress her shortly after her death. In the few hours before you call the funeral home there will be no swelling, no smell or "blackening" of the body. You are not going to keep her there for days, only a few hours.

People across the country are having in home funerals and visitations and are very pleased that they have done it. Google information about in home funerals for more information and guidance.

I am sorry to say, your mother will die. Because of her age it will be sooner than most of us. Whether or not you feed her and exercise her, she will die and in the not too distant future. Most of us don't live to be 100 and even fewer of us live past it. How lucky she has been. How fortunate you all have been to have her this long. I certainly understand why you don't want to let the remaining time she has left with her family to be unhappy, painful, stressful and alone.

Section III: Food And Water

It's Okay Not To Eat

Months before death from disease and often years before death from simply old age, a person's eating habits change. They gradually begin eating less and less. Food is what keeps our body going. It is where we get our energy and grounding. If the body is preparing to die it will naturally cut back on what it eats. Beginning months before death a person will stop eating meat, then it becomes fruits and vegetables, then soft food. By the weeks before death a person is barely eating anything. Ice cream and liquids are often the best they can do. Generally, in the days before death, a person will not be able to eat anything including even water. All of this is part of the normal way a body dies.

One of the hardest things for people to understand is that when a person has entered the dying process it is okay not to eat; that literally the person reaches a point where they CAN'T eat. They just can't do it even when they want to.

For us, the people involved with a loved one approaching death, our heart tells us that if they would just eat everything would be better. We know they have to eat to live so if we "make" them eat they will live. There are several factors at work here, and a big factor is whether the person eats or not the disease, which can't be fixed, will still progress and the person will die. Eating will not make things better. In fact artificial feeding (feeding tubes, a gastrostomy) may make matters worse, creating more complications than benefit.

When addressing the not eating, not enough calories for maintenance that occurs naturally as end of life approaches, my recommendation is to ALWAYS OFFER FOOD, just don't force the food. Offer favorites, offer high calorie high protein liquid supplements, offer water but accept what is or is not eaten.

Nothing bad is happening at this time in the dying process. What is happening is part of the normal, natural way that people die. It is us, the watchers, the ones who don't want our loved one to leave us, who don't understand the natural dying process that have a new challenge. We are the ones who have to learn that the body of the person that is dying will stop eating and processing nutrients and that the disease will continue to progress no matter how much we intervene.

It's Okay Not To Drink Water

On our journey toward physical death, as the body stops eating food, it also stops drinking water. We all recognize the body's need for hydration (water) to live and as our loved one stops drinking water we tend to panic and think we should have IV fluids (water given through a needle and tubing in the arm) to keep the body at least comfortable if not nourished.

When a person has entered the dying process their body begins letting go of its hold on the physical, first letting go of food, then letting go of water. The entire physical body is shutting down. As it shuts down, it stops functioning normally. The kidneys that process liquids are not performing their job, so if you begin IV fluids often times the fluid stays trapped in the cells of the body and the lungs, causing increased discomfort.

The dying body doesn't want nutrition or hydration (food or water). When a person has entered the dying process and they are not eating any food and not drinking sufficient liquid to keep them hydrated they are days to a week or so from death. From a medical standpoint, the calcium in their blood will begin to rise because there is not enough water in the body to operate efficiently. When the calcium gets high enough a person just goes to sleep and doesn't wake up. If left to its own devices the body itself gives comfort in sleep. A sleep that allows us to leave this world and begin our new journey. This is the normal, natural way to die.

Is It A Choice To Not Eat?

QUESTION: *Is a diagnosis of "Failure to Thrive" a choice on the part of the patient when they consciously refuse to eat?*

I'm not sure that most people "consciously" refuse to eat. We tend to think the elderly and those very sick are making a choice, generally they are not. Their body is shutting down and the body, not the personality, just can't eat anymore. Remember, it is food that holds us on this planet and if the body is preparing to die, to let go, it will gradually stop eating. No choice is involved here.

There are some people (few, but some) who consciously decide to stop eating so that they can die: People with a poor prognosis, a life threatening illness, people in pain with no cure in sight, people who feel not eating is the only control they now have in their life. These people will sometimes make the choice to not eat. If we don't eat we will die.

What do we do when a person with a life threatening illness is not eating? We always, always offer food. My suggestion is if a person has been told they can't be fixed and they are entering the dying process, don't force them to eat. Offer food, but don't go the artificial feeding path. Offer them high protein snacks (4-6 a day) also offer them 4 ounces of a liquid protein supplement every 2 hours. The operative word here is offer. You will not stop the non eating progression but you may buy a bit of time and energy.

The person will die from the disease progression; not because they didn't get enough calories. We tend to think a person with a life threatening illness who doesn't eat dies of starvation when in reality, a person dies from the disease. Not eating is an offshoot of the disease. Yes, most people do not take enough calories for maintaining a body as they approach death from disease or old age. What we need to know is that not eating is part of how people die a gradual death.

By artificially feeding them with TPN or tube feedings we do not reverse the terminal disease progression; we don't stop it or even slow it down. The person will die either way. It is just that they will die having had one more medical procedure, one more disruption to their body, generally with more discomfort.

Feeding Tube?

QUESTION: *If a family member suffers a stroke what is the right decision about whether to use a feeding tube?*

I think it depends on what a person's mind and body are like after the stroke. How severe is the damage? What is the potential for rehabilitation? Quality of living is what would influence my decision about whether to have a feeding tube.

If I had a stroke and some of my body functions were impaired, but I could think, communicate, read, understand, laugh, get out of bed, and leave the house, but I had difficulty swallowing to the point of choking, I would probably choose a feeding tube.

If I couldn't do any of those things; required someone to address my bodily functions for me, had to leave my home and be cared for in a facility, couldn't get out of bed, and most of all did not have my mental alertness and awareness, then no feeding tube for me.

The bottom line in making feeding tube decisions is quality of life. What kind of living is the nourishment going to sustain? Are we putting the person through the discomfort of creating an artificial hole in their stomach, to then develop a routine for having liquid nourishment flowing into that stomach, just so the physical body will continue breathing? Or are we providing nourishment so the person can ENJOY the life the food is providing?

Too often we are offered life sustaining options without considering what kind of life we are sustaining. Just because we can do a medical procedure does not mean it is necessarily in our best interest to have it done. This applies to many medical options that are offered today.

Section IV: Pain At End Of Life

Medications

QUESTION: *Will you talk about sedation at the end of life?*

There is a misconception that dying is painful, therefore pain medicine/narcotics should be used routinely in the last days to weeks of life. We need to add to that discussion tranquilizers (to calm) and sedatives (to induce sleep).

Let's begin with pain when dying. Dying does not cause pain; disease causes pain. Not all diseases create pain so we need to look at a person's disease history to determine if we are witnessing actual physical pain, mild flu-like discomfort or our own fears as we watch the labor of dying.

If physical pain has been a part of the disease process, then pain medicine in quantities to create comfort need to be administered around the clock, 24/7, until death has occurred. Pharmacologically speaking, there is no reason for anyone to die in physical pain today. People die in pain today because of ignorance, fear, and lack of communication and understanding on the part of caregivers, physicians and significant others.

If physical pain has not been an issue in the disease history then generally the physical sensations will be similar to flu-like heaviness, that ache all over sensation. If you had the flu you would not take a narcotic. You would take a couple of Ibuprofen. So it is when a person is dying. If pain has not been an issue in the disease process (this is the key point I am making here: when pain has not been part of the disease) then the person doesn't need a narcotic. You can give them an analgesic which will provide comfort. Giving narcotics for respiratory distress is another whole issue and can be very appropriate and comforting.

Restlessness is also a natural part of the dying process. It can be due to lack of oxygen but generally it is the dying person's subconscious fear of approaching death, of entering an unknown experience. If the restlessness is mild, picking the clothes or random hand movements, nothing needs to be done medically. If the restlessness becomes agitation, to the point you are concerned the person will fall out of bed or otherwise will hurt themselves, then a mild medication is very appropriate; Haldol and Ativan both work very well.

Sedatives generally aren't necessary as death approaches. There may be a semantics issue here between tranquilizer and sedative. I am using sedative to mean sleep inducement. Sleep comes naturally in the dying process. It gradually increases over three to four months before death actually occurs. Most people naturally sleep (are non responsive) in the hours to even days before death. We generally don't go from saying something very profound to those at our bedside to taking our last breath. That scenario is only in the movies. When we are dying a gradual death from disease or old age, most of us are asleep, even though we may be moving and muttering, in the last days to moments of our life.

What I really believe is that most often the issue of pain during the dying process is more of a concern for us the watchers (that includes doctors and nurses as well as family and significant others) because we are afraid and not understanding what is happening and less a physical reality of the dying person. We bring our fears, our role models, our stereotypes, our imagination, and our culture to the bedside and that natural, normal labor we are watching is then translated into the belief that physical pain is occurring.

Morphine

QUESTION: *Talk about the use of morphine "to ease the pain that is often present as a person approaches death."*

First I will say there is not always pain as death nears. Most people don't know this. Most of us think when we are dying we will have pain. Not true. Dying is not the source of pain; disease is the source of pain and not all diseases cause pain. There are many diseases that can't be fixed; that cause the body to stop working, stop living, but don't do it in a painful way. There are other diseases that cause a great deal of pain and discomfort.

With today's medical advances there is no reason for anyone to die in pain. There are many, many different pain medications to choose from. Generally, the intensity of the pain the disease is creating and the disease itself will depend upon which medication is used.

There are non narcotic drugs that can be very effective and there are patches that are put on the skin that can be effective but take longer to regulate. There are pills, liquids, creams, intravenous, and suppositories; all different forms of pain medication.

Morphine is a frequently used narcotic to relieve most types of end of life pain but it has a fearful reputation. Most people hear the word morphine and immediately think of addiction and overdose. If there was no pain in your body and you started taking morphine, yes, you would become addicted and may even overdose; BUT for someone who has pain in their body, the morphine will work on the pain, not the healthy body.

There is a thin line in everyone's body between pain and no pain. If the pain is so severe that non narcotic medication does not reduce or eliminate it, then it is appropriate to use a narcotic without the fear of addiction or overdose. When you find the line between pain and no pain (which may take several days of dosage adjustments) then a person can generally be alert and comfortable.

If for some reason comfort cannot be achieved, a person can be given a dosage of morphine that is high enough to induce sleep but not death. The person will sleep and therefore not be aware of the pain until the body is ready to die. The medical term for this is Palliative Sedation. At no time is morphine used with the intent to end life.

In managing severe, terminal pain we need to be aware that the pain medication does not eliminate the pain. It just covers it up. What is causing the pain is still and will always be there. Because we are just covering it up, the "cover" must be kept on it continually. That means the medication is taken around the clock.

A mistake that often occurs is that we take the medicine until we aren't hurting and then stop taking it. We think "I'll take the pills when the pain comes back." With terminal pain if you wait until you are hurting before you take the medicine you will always be playing catch up and not be truly comfortable.

Pain management at end of life is an entire workshop of information; in fact several workshops. I have just touched on a few basic points to consider. Read my booklet, Pain At End of Life, for more information.

Lack Of Knowledge

I received the following comment on my blog. "They are overmedicating Mom" (The family said of hospice professionals). "Following a brief rally, she slept most of the time and died within a week. Her sons concluded she was being overmedicated with pain medication; with less medication, she would wake up and be alert again. They wanted Mom back, understandably, but that was not to be and it was not because of the pain medication…she was dying."

You are correct in your assessment, Mom probably did not die because she was over medicated. The family concerns you mention are so often exactly what people believe; "If Mom didn't have the pain medicine she could have talked with them, would have been alert and might not have died when she did".

What most people don't know is that months before death from disease or old age, the dying process begins. A person begins eating less and less, sleeping more and more, withdrawing inward, and talking less and less.

In the weeks before death, a person is asleep more than awake, eating almost nothing and generally does not initiate conversation. They will respond when spoken to, although often they are confused.

In the days to hours before death, a person is generally non responsive, meaning they may be moving and talking but not making sense and not responding to the world around them. This is the normal progression of gradual dying from disease or old age.

How much medication a person has is not the issue here. This progression will occur with or without medication. Withholding the medication will not have the patient waking up and talking if indeed death is days to hours away.

Withholding the medication will leave the patient less comfortable, overly agitated, restless, and possibly with aggravated air hunger (difficulty breathing).

Know that it is harder to watch a loved one dying than it is to die. The person dying is so withdrawn and removed from their body in the days to hours before death that they are not experiencing their body and its sensations in the same manner as a healthy person.

Did Morphine Kill?

QUESTION: *I have a man that regrets giving his father morphine for pain at the end. His father had cancer all over. What would you say to him to make him understand that he did not kill his father? After his father passed a family member made a comment that he gave morphine until his father died.*

The use of Morphine is one of the most misunderstood practices I encounter with families and end of life issues. Our society is so drug conscious we tend to equate any use as misuse.

First, let's understand end of life pain. Dying is not painful, disease causes pain. If pain has not been an issue in the person's disease history, then just because death is approaching does not mean the person is in pain. We do not need to use a narcotic for comfort. Ibuprofen is my drug of choice.

If pain has been an issue during the disease process, then we certainly want to continue to provide adequate pain management until the last breath is taken. Just because a person is non-responsive (which most people are before death) does not mean that pain is not there. We also need to know that whatever was causing the pain is not removed by the narcotic. The narcotic just covers up the pain. We must keep the cover on. In end of life pain management we also need to know that the use of narcotics over time tends to require increasing the amount of the narcotic.

Now let's address the major concern---hastening death with the administration of morphine (or any narcotic). When a person is days to hours before death, their body is shutting down. Nothing works right. Circulation, the blood flowing through the body, is slower and less effective (this is what the bluish color to the hands and feet shows). When you give any medication at that time, it does not get absorbed and become effective in the same way it would in a body that's functioning normally. This is why giving pain medicine to someone who is actively dying is rarely the cause of death.

This father had "cancer all over." I believe that means he had the potential for pain, lots of pain, in his disease progression. Morphine given continually is a must to keep this man relaxed and relatively comfortable. The morphine did not kill him; it allowed him to leave this world more gently than if he were suffering physically.

Here is a controversial thought. What if the morphine had killed his father? He had a terminal illness. In fact, his father was actually in the dying process. There was no reversing what was physically happening. Death was coming. What if hours of life (a few hours) could be extended by withholding the pain medicine? The result would be physical pain causing agitation and extreme discomfort, even though the body is non-responsive. By continuing to give the morphine, the last hours could be relaxed and relatively comfortable. Either way the person, as death approaches, is non-responsive. The misconception is that by withholding the narcotic the person would be alert and interactive. That is not the case. Either way the person will be non-responsive. It is just that in one scenario the person is hurting and in the other they are not. Which would you want?

The Patch

QUESTION: *"The effectiveness of liquid morphine & Ativan seemed inadequate. The 'active dying' process took six days---no food, no water, and it seemed her body began to decay before our eyes. Even the hospice nurses were somewhat surprised at her strength. We were able to give her wonderful care at home, and hospice was a valuable resource, but we were strongly opposed to the use of a narcotic patch for additional comfort care. Finally we did start the patches, and wished they could have been started sooner. We still struggle with the memory of those final days, and the periodic suffering she experienced.*

There are several areas in the above comment I am going to address: comfort management, use of a transdermal patch, the normal dying process and being at the bedside watching someone we care about die.

Comfort management: Pain is unique to each individual. There is no one dose, one kind, one method that fits all. Unlike the old adage, "Take two aspirin and call me in the morning", end of life pain management requires time and experimentation to reach a comfort level. Closeness to death itself also affects how medications will be responded to. The closer to death the less circulation there is to distribute the medication throughout the body.

Use of a transdermal patch: A patch is pain medicine commercially put into patch form and applied directly to the skin. Some end of life care professionals like and use the patch system, others do not. I personally do not use the patch if the person is within days of death for a couple of reasons.

Early in the disease process a patch can be an excellent source of pain relief but when very close to death, circulation is poor so absorption is poor. Mainly, a patch is a specific dosage for a specific time period and what is needed, as death approaches is the ability to regulate the dosage and time frame to each individual. Patches and time release medications do not allow that latitude.

If the person is non responsive and unable to swallow but is agitated and pain has been a part of their disease process, then medication can be given rectally or made into a creme and rubbed onto the skin. Generally there is no need for invasive injections or IV medications.

The dying process: In the one to three week time period before death a person enters what I refer to as labor. That labor is harder on us the watchers than it is on the person who is actively dying. The person who is dying is so removed from their body that they are not experiencing it in the same way we the watchers are perceiving.

In those days to weeks before death, the person is not eating or drinking or they are taking so little fluids we believe they can't possibly be comfortable. This is the time the body is shutting down, letting go of its hold on this life, dying. No food or water in the last days of life is perfectly normal. That is how we die. It is not uncomfortable or painful to not eat or drink at this stage. It is actually uncomfortable and disruptive for the dying person if we force food and water in the days to weeks before death.

This is a short explanation about a complicated subject. Watching someone we care about in the dying process is frightening, stressful and generally misunderstood. Knowledge reduces fear, but it is generally after the fact that we begin processing and asking questions. Having someone close to us in the dying process is so very sad but with a bit of knowledge it doesn't have to be a bad experience.

Just Because They Are Dying

QUESTION: *Talk about a chemical straight jacket. My mother is a dementia patient in a memory unit. Hospice now. They are giving increased Ativan & morphine to "keep her comfortable". We are in very last days now. Don't want her to suffer, but somehow this seems wrong.*

I have not heard the words "chemical straight jacket" before but I see the implication---controlling patient movements with drugs rather than physical restraints. Nursing facility regulations are very strict now about physically restraining agitated patients, medications not so much, if you can justify the reason.

I do not think there is a need for narcotics just because death is approaching. Dying is not painful. Disease causes pain. Dementia does not cause pain unless the person is actively hurting themselves or there is another physical condition that causes pain.

Part of the natural dying process is restlessness. There is a picking of the clothes and bed linen. There is an agitation of just not being settled, tossing, and turning. If that restlessness is not causing harm or putting the patient at physical risk, then I do not feel medications are necessary. If the restlessness puts the patient in harms way (falling out of bed, injuring themselves) then Ativan or some relaxant seems appropriate.

Increased use of narcotics and relaxants as end of life approaches has become quite common in the end of life arena---much to my concern. Why is this happening? One: end of life has become more medicalized, more intertwined with the medical system. We seem to have forgotten that dying is not a medical event. It is a social, communal event. Two: I think there is a lack of understanding of the dying process. What is natural versus what is pathological (even among medical professionals). With this lack of understanding is the deep desire to keep a person comfortable, to help them approach death in as comfortable a way as possible; not ending life but providing comfort until death comes. I think this is admirable but based in lack of knowledge. Our end of life professionals need to know better.

When a person is in the labor of dying and pain is not a part of the disease process, we do not need to begin a pain management protocol just because the person is dying.

Help Me Die

QUESTION: *Dying "euthanized" or given fairly heavy duty morphine drips to allow "dying in peace". I've also seen doctors recommend it to "hasten" the painful process of dying. Most people do not believe that death is not painful. I've also seen patients who ask for morphine to hasten the process. That's my question... should a dying person be offered that choice and would it be considered medically legal?*

I don't think offering a patient the choice of receiving a dosage of medication that will end life is legal. Look at all the discussion and controversy about physician-assisted death which is legal in several states but still causes much descent.

As health caregivers our job is to provide care prescribed by the attending physician --not to make major medical decisions on our own for the patient. We provide care, not prescribe it. It is certainly not within our role to act if a person, in the pain of the moment, wants help in ending their life. In the "pain of the moment" are the operative words here. I cannot tell you the number of times I have heard that plea in the throes of pain, and the relief when that pain subsides and life continues.

Now let's talk about the pain of dying. In my experience and observations dying is not painful. DISEASE causes pain. To the observer the labor in the days before death can look painful: the restlessness, the congestion, the aggravated breathing, the facial expressions and the body coloring (mottled, ashen).

The body is not functioning in a "normal" manner. The systems are shutting down, as is thinking, interacting, reacting, and responding. When pain is not part of the disease process (and there are alot of diseases that people die from that do not cause pain) it is the people watching that tend to translate what they are watching into pain. Our fear of what we are seeing, sees pain. I do not see it as our place to make the choice to end a person's life because of our perceptions of suffering.

In the months before death occurs pain is at its highest. Why? Because that is when we are alert and aware and when our fears and emotions tend to escalate the pain. I certainly am not saying the pain isn't real---it is very real. I am saying that the flame is higher because of our emotions. As death gets closer and we begin disconnecting from this reality the emotions play less of a part in the pain. In the days before death we are generally unresponsive and only our body language and those around us with their perceptions show our pain.

If pain has been a part of the disease process, always give the pain medicine up to the moment of death. Increase the dosage with a physician's order if restlessness is intense. Our goal is always comfort but not death. Often healthcare workers fear that they have "killed" a patient if death comes within minutes after giving the pain medicine. That is probably not the cause of death. If death occurred that soon after the medication was given, the circulation which carries the medicine through the blood stream was so diminished that a regular dosage would have no effect.

"Should they be offered the choice?" In a way, yes, I think a person should be offered the choice of how they want their life to end. That talk needs to be at the beginning of the disease process. At a time when how a person wants to live their life and how they want their last months, weeks, days and hours to be is not colored by the withdrawal, the disconnect from reality, and the pressure of pain.

This is why Advanced Directives are so important. They describe how we want to live until we are dead. "Medicate me as much as possible if pain is part of my disease" is an appropriate addition to an Advanced Directive.

As we lay dying, days to hours before our body succumbs to the inevitable, we will be unable to make decisions for ourselves. HOWEVER, I strongly believe that we do not want a practice developed that puts the decision to end our life in the hands of others---no matter how much we plead at the time.

Guidelines

There is so much confusion and fear regarding end of life pain medicines, morphine in particular, that I am addressing what I consider major issues. I have made the list simple, short, and to the point so that you can use this as a guideline when your loved one is receiving a narcotic as the end of their life approaches.

- To be effective, pain medicine needs to be given on a regular, around the clock, schedule.
- Over time the original dosage may have to be increased.
- Everyone's pain is different so everyone's pain medicine and amount will be different.
- There is no standardized medicine dosage for pain. It takes time to find the correct pain medicine and the correct amount.
- Most medicines given by mouth can be given rectally. Some pain medicines can be made into creams and rubbed on the skin.
- Generally there isn't a need for needles in end of life pain management.
- Pain doesn't stop when a person is non-responsive. Continue the pain management schedule until death.

I am adding an additional caveat to the above knowledge: Dying is not painful. Disease causes pain. If pain has not been an issue during the disease process then just because a person is actively dying does not mean they are in pain. If pain has been an issue during the disease process, that pain is present to the last breath.

Often dying looks painful to the people watching. Dying is a struggle to get out of the body. There are sounds that ordinarily would indicate discomfort but, when a person is actively dying, those sounds are part of the struggle.

Just as the little chick works to get out of its shell, a person works to get out of their body. It takes effort to release from our body. That includes rattling and gasping sounds, twitching, random hand and leg movements, picking the air, facial grimaces, and talking that doesn't make sense. All of this is part of the natural struggle to get out of the body. Nothing bad is happening, nothing pathological. This is how people and other animals die.

What I have described in the paragraph above is generally interpreted as an expression of pain unless someone tells the watchers differently. That is where knowledge of end of life and the dying process comes in; that is where health care professionals can give important guidance IF they, themselves, understand the normal, natural way people die. Sad to say, all too often, even health care professionals do not know.

Section V: Children

Coping

QUESTION: *Talk about coping over the years after the loss of a child.*

Children are our legacy to the world. They are a piece of ourselves. They are what we leave behind when we die. Our children certainly are not supposed to die before we do.

How do we cope with our grief over the death of our child? With strength, perseverance, gratitude and time.

Strength to get out of bed and put one foot in front of the other to get through each day. Strength to figure out how to go on living.

Perseverance to cry the tears, scream the screams, rage with the anger and then move forward in the day knowing the tears, screams and rage will come again and again and still we move forward.

Gratitude for the gift the child gave us by being in our life for however long it was. Better to have had the gift for a short time than never at all. Gratitude for the love and joy of being a parent.

And time--time gradually fills in the space between the pain. We don't heal or recover or even understand why our loved one is gone from us. Time simply makes life a bit more bearable as we live with our loss.

Death Has No Age Limit

QUESTION: *Please talk about unexpected youth death.*

In our minds we understand that as sad as it is when an older adult dies, they have lived their life and death comes to us all. Even when a young or middle aged adult dies, we are shocked, saddened but think they had their chance at living. When a peer dies, someone our own age, we experience shock in our grieving as death brushes past us too close for comfort. BUT when a young person, a child or a teen, dies our world is shaken to its core. It seems that a law has been broken.

The young are not supposed to die. They are our future. They have not had a chance to live, to experience, to grow old. For parents, their legacy is taken away. The opportunity to see themselves in their child is stolen. For parents, no matter the age of the child, but even more so with the young, a piece of themselves dies also.

I cannot think of deeper grief than the grief for a child lost. For some, they never find a way to go on living. Grief for all of us is not about getting over, recovering or even healing. All of us who lose someone have to learn how to live with our grief. Time mostly lessens the external pain but inwardly we must find life and living, a reason to continue. It is harder for us to find our way forward when we experience the death of our child.

For many, finding a cause, a purpose in memory of our child, gives direction to an emptier life. It helps to find something to keep their name, their memory, alive. Foundations, alerts, ribbons can be a channel for our grief. Channel the pain into a positive direction. Giving help and assistance to others in the name of our precious child doesn't lessen our feelings of loss, but it can bring something positive into our lives when all we feel is the negative. Something as simple as planting a tree and watching it grow can bring a bit of comfort in what feels like a comfortless world.

I know the question asked here was about the unexpected death of a child and my response applies to all deaths of children, gradual or fast. I think even if a child is ill (for that matter even adults) we are never prepared for the death. They are all basically unexpected. Many of us just can't come to the realization that death is coming no matter how much we fight, cry, close our eyes and deny it. Dying has no age limit. Dying is very much a part of living.

Suicide

Dear Barbara, A friend of mine had a child commit suicide. Do you have reference material that I might use to help my friend.

I do not have any reference material specifically for those people left behind following a suicide. Google might give you some information.

My two cents--- part of normal grief is all the questions we will never have answers to, the whys and what ifs? With suicide those questions are tenfold. With a child's suicide those questions are a million fold.

Blame is a feeling and series of thoughts we also have surrounding suicide; blaming others, blaming the person that died, and blaming ourselves. "If we had done things differently this life would not have been taken" is paramount in our mind.

As a society, and often through religion, we place guilt and shame, not only toward the person that has taken their life but on the family and significant others as well. This stigma adds to the grief we are feeling and experiencing.

All this information will really not affect the intense grief and many emotions that make up the grief your friend feels. A suicide takes normal grieving to a whole different level. No answers will be found, no understanding will make any sense. I can just say that for some people, children included, life is too difficult to let it play itself out to a natural ending.

There are no words, no prayers, no pills that can ease the pain of loss, guilt, recriminations and confusion that come with suicide, particularly the suicide of a child. Being a friend who cares, who is there, a presence, is of greatest value for the griever.

Adult Children

QUESTION: *I have a twenty-three year old daughter that has a chronic illness. She says she is tired of fighting. I don't want to lose her. I am lost.*

Having our children hurt and struggling in life can be devastating for us as parents. There is such a helpless and even hopeless feeling in watching our adult children with their challenges. When they were little we could kiss the hurt and make it better—-now what do we do? Kisses aren't enough.

As a parent of adult children, I have found that one of the hardest parts of our relationship is to support them in their choice when I would have chosen something different for them. I have learned the hard way that I can offer ideas but then must be quiet and let them make their own choices. They, and I, have to live with the consequences of those choices. Oh so tough for a parent to do. When it comes to life threatening situations we can still only offer our ideas, support, and love.

My suggestion is to keep her talking. Talk about how hard it is to live being sick. Help her find joy in each day (even if the joy is so small she can barely find it). Help her avoid being isolated from others (too much time alone leads to dwelling on how hard life is, instead of finding good in the day that you have).

For you, find a friend to share your feelings with, one who will listen to you as you share your fears and frustrations. In helping your daughter find joy, you will also find it.

Remember LIFE is a terminal illness. We are, all of us, dying each day. It is what we DO with each individual day that has the value, not how many days we accumulate on this planet.

Miscarriage-Stillborn

October 15 was National Pregnancy and Infant Loss Remembrance Day. I've been asked to write about the grief experienced with the loss of a baby through miscarriage or stillbirth. I am not an expert in this kind of grief, I can only share what I have learned along life's way.

In the late 1960's I was five and a half months pregnant with twins when I was told quite bluntly, "You have twins. I know one is dead but I am not sure about the other. It is probably dead too. You will just have to wait and see how this plays out." I was to stay pregnant until I went into natural labor. I carried those little girls for a month inside of my body knowing they were dead. Here is what I learned from that experience.

For that month I was numb. I cried and I talked about what the doctor had said, I was angry at how casually he told me (over the phone) but basically I was shut down. I went about my daily routine of being a stay at home mom of two children, three and five years old.

My husband and I didn't talk about it after the first round of tears and dismay. My best friend was pregnant also and where we had shared our pregnancies now it was silent between us on that subject--sadness, but "how can you have a healthy pregnancy and I don't" thoughts were also there. I knew that the rest of my family supported and cared for me but there was a silence there also. No one knew what to say to me, so they didn't say anything. There was an elephant in the room and I was it, almost literally and definitely metaphorically.

I accidentally fell down which brought on labor. After the birth, which I slept through thanks to pharmaceuticals, I was placed in a double room at the end of the hall on the maternity floor of the hospital. My roommate had given birth to a stillborn baby. The curtain between the beds was drawn the entire time; we never talked. Rarely did the staff come into our room. We were isolated, we were alone but we could hear the laughter in the other rooms and, hardest of all, we could hear babies crying.

When I got home life returned to "normal". There was no talk about what had happened, or about loss and grief. It was as if those little girls had never happened. To make it real I gave them names and placed those names in our family Bible. When my friend had her baby it was a challenge to walk to her house and hold her baby. We acknowledged how uncomfortable it was and then didn't talk about it ever again. Life moved on.

A little over a year later I had another child, a healthy, beautiful little girl. I worried throughout the entire pregnancy (now I knew things could go wrong, loss could occur beyond my control). Once Jackie was born I became an overprotective, nervous mom. I was afraid something would happen to her. But there was also value and appreciation in being a mom that I hadn't had before. I knew in my core now how fragile motherhood could be.

I am sharing this story because I don't think I am any different than other women in how I reacted to the loss of a child before it had even been born. The grief of my lost babies was never acknowledged. I lived as if nothing had happened. But feelings get expressed in other ways if we don't deal with them straight on. My grief came out in my overprotectiveness and an intense search for meaning to life. In hindsight I can see that search has lead me to where I am today.

I was in a workshop with Elizabeth Kuebler Ross ten years later and when she talked about miscarriages and stillborn experiences I sobbed for the first time for those little girls, for the life they didn't have, for my fear, my isolation. She gave me permission to recognize the experience as relevant, to see that loss as life changing, and to feel the pain of silence that I had carried all that time.

Today we are better at recognizing the legitimacy of the loss and the ensuing grief that comes with miscarriages and stillborn children. There are resources available, counseling sessions and support groups. We have some hospices that provide services that begin when the baby is recognized as being dead or will be dead upon birth. Babies are dressed, pictures taken, love, conversations and holding are encouraged. Families are supported and guided through this experience as well as the mother. Hopefully the isolation and silence has been broken.

Section VI: Meaning

Faith

QUESTION: *Where do you mention one's faith in your materials? Please discuss.*

The definition of the word faith from the Free Merriam-Webster dictionary is:

(1) : fidelity to one's promises (2) : sincerity of intentions. 2 a (1) : belief and trust in and loyalty to God (2) : belief in the traditional doctrines of a religion. b (1) : firm belief in something for which there is no proof (2) : complete trust.

Approaching the end of our life generally promotes questions and searching about purpose, meaning and the direction our life has taken. Any of the above definitions for faith apply to our end of life search. These thoughts may not be shared with anyone but I believe we ask ourselves questions like: What have I done? Who have I touched? What has this life been about? What is my belief about an after life? And, if a belief in God has been a part of our life, have I lived up to the expectations I believe are a part of a relationship with God?

Because our relationship with God, or absence of a relationship with God, is very personal it is not up to outsiders to try to influence that relationship unless asked. The operative words here are "unless asked". Facing the end of life is not the time for conversions or saving, again, unless asked.

Because on many levels we are asking meaningful questions about the course our life has taken, major spiritual work is being done. It is work that is done by only one, the person approaching death. As the dying process progresses, withdrawal from this world reaches a place of introspection.

It appears people are merely sleeping when really they are doing perhaps the most important work of their lives---figuring out what their life has been about. It is solitary work done by the person approaching death.

I don't mention spiritual beliefs in my materials because I feel approaching the end of our life is a personal search and not a place for others to share their beliefs unless, of course, we are asked.

With people of the same religion, same beliefs, such as with members of a church, synagogue, mosque, shrine, temple, etc. I believe that in the months before death spiritual conversations are helpful, again, if they are initiated by the person facing death. Some people welcome conversations, others prefer to find answers from within.

We must always respect a person's choices. Remember, we approach this final challenge in our life in the same manner we have approached all of our challenges. If a belief in God and/or a specific religion was not a part of living our life, our beliefs will probably not change now. I will add that sometimes we will return to the religion and belief we had when we were younger but this doesn't seem to happen enough to really count on it.

There are many paths to self discovery; religions are one path. My goal in presenting my materials is to walk a broader path presenting spirituality but not under the name of a specific ideology in the hopes that each of us, regardless of our beliefs, may experience compassionate end of life care.

Non Existance

QUESTION: *Talk about the concept of "not existing" any longer. I believe this is the fear people may fear and not the unknown. If there was something "to be known" by one's belief then that would suffice. Extinction is another concept that an atheist may wrestle with. Your comments here are appreciated.*

This is a tough one to answer because each individual's personality enters into what we think about these profound ideas.

I wonder if we can even conceive of not existing. Can we imagine what that would be like? We have our bodies that age and change but there is that "voice" (what I refer to as "the driver") that is inside of us, thinking, feeling, perceiving, reacting all the time. It doesn't seem to age. It just IS us. I'm not sure we can comprehend not having that part of us.

Religions imply that the IS of us lives on. Reincarnation implies that also. We interpret both of those philosophies to mean that the IS that is us continues just in a different way. No extinction here and a lot of comfort.

Does the idea of not existing tie into the fear of the unknown? We don't really know what happens to the IS of us after our body dies. There are so many stories about communication after the physical body stops; stories of Near Death Experiences, stories from world cultures, and ancient religions. These different beliefs and sharing instill in us a question; that question being "do we really cease to exist when the physical body stops?" That one question, with no definitive answer, makes a belief in non-existence suspect.

Different religions teach different ideas of what happens after breathing stops and we are dead-- teaching about a life after death. Even with those teachings ingrained in our belief system, we really don't know for sure. Therein lies the unknown and the fear that we all will wrestle with as we approach death.

As for atheists and those religions that teach that we only live on in other's memories, I think the fear of dying is the same as those with a belief in an after life. For all of us it is all about "life as we know it is going to be over, I don't want it to be over, and what happens to me when it is?"

There Are No Accidents

QUESTION: *How could God let my child die. How could God let teenagers, shoot other teenagers. I am losing any faith I ever had as I watch this world full of violence.*

I am so sorry your child died. I am so sorry other children are dying. I am so sorry that anyone we love and are close to dies. I can think of no grief stronger than the grief that comes with the death of a child. The grief from a violent death is compounded a million fold. There are no words that I or anyone can say that will make sense of your loss or make you feel better. Even when I say that time will ease, but not erase the pain, it will be hard for you to believe me.

It doesn't make sense that a child's time on earth can be over when it seems it hasn't begun. These and thousands of questions like them, are what we ask when death comes to someone we love. It will never be okay for our children, or our parents, or our friends to die, no matter what ages. It will never be acceptable, under any circumstances, for anyone to die violently. How do we live with the unacceptable?

I am going to share with you the idea that gets me through the night; an idea that makes sense to me, even though it does not lessen the pain ---as I said, nothing lessens the pain of loss.

Death is not accidental. We die when it is our time to die, no sooner, no later. Everything happens for a reason. We, the survivors, most often just don't understand the reason. These two ideas make sense to me but that doesn't make it any easier to accept when someone is dying.

I believe we live until our work here is finished. Who is to say we haven't done what we came here to do in 3 months, in 10 years or in 80 years?

To believe that death is not accidental, that there comes a time when a person's work in life is finished, no matter the age, is an act of faith. Faith in the idea that I can only perceive and understand a small portion of this vast experience called life. Faith that most of what occurs round and about me I will not understand. Faith that the best I can do is believe that all is as it should be. Faith that as overwhelming as my grief is, it is another life experience for me to grow through.